iCare

Express

Photozig, Inc.

iCare Express:

iCare® Express is part of an informative program developed by Photozig, Inc. in collaboration with Stanford University, Alzheimer's Association, and other organizations, which was funded by the National Institute on Aging (part of the National Institutes of Health), and specifically created for caregivers of individuals with dementia or memory loss.

The educational iCare program describes the skills on how to cope with caregiving, reduce related distress, and improve the quality of life of caregivers and loved ones.

For additional information, please go to the iCare web site at: **www.icarefamily.com**

Contact Us:

Any questions about the iCare project should be addressed to the project staff at Photozig, Inc:

icare@photozig.com

www.icarefamily.com

Important Notes:

The instructions and advice presented in this publication are in no way intended as a substitute for professional medical judgment and assistance. It is not intended to treat any medical or psychological problems. This publication is an educational tool only, to help you learn more about dementia and to give you information about common ways to cope with related problems. Not all of the information provided is suitable for everyone, and we do not guarantee or promise that the techniques illustrated in this publication will be helpful to every individual caregiver who watches this DVD or reads/uses this handbook. For example, the problems you are confronted with may be different from the ones presented here, or you may have so many problems that you are overwhelmed and in need of professional assistance in order to cope effectively with your situation. Individuals with medical conditions should not use the "Deep Breathing" or any of the techniques presented here for stress management without their doctor's advice and approval. To reduce the risk of injury, consult your doctor before beginning this or any caregiver program. The instructions and advice presented here are in no way intended as a substitute for family counseling, psychotherapy, or any form of medical treatment.

Acknowledgments:

This project is supported by Award Number R44AG032762 from the National Institute on Aging. The content is solely the responsibility of the authors and does not necessarily represent the official views of the National Institute on Aging or the National Institutes of Health.

Credits

Research Team

Bruno Kajiyama, MS
Principal Investigator, Photozig, Inc.

Dolores Gallagher-Thompson, PhD, ABPP
Co-Principal Investigator
Stanford University School of Medicine

Larry Thompson, PhD
Co-Principal Investigator
Stanford University School of Medicine

Photozig Healthcare Research

Irene Rivera-Valverde, BA, MFTT
John Di Mario, BS
Marian Tzuang, MSW
Mio Yamashita, MA, ATR, MFT
Tamiko Eto-Iwase, MA

Advisory Committee

David Coon, PhD
Arizona State University

Elizabeth Edgerly, PhD
Alzheimer's Association of Northern California & Northern Nevada

Ladson Hinton, MD
UC Davis Medical School & UC Davis Alzheimer's Disease Center

Suzann Ogland-Hand, PhD
Pine Rest Christian Mental Health Service

For further information, please visit **www.icarefamily.com**

We would like to thank all organizations that supported this project, including the National Institutes of Health (NIH), Alzheimer's Association, NASA, and Stanford University.

This research was substantially supported by grant R44AG032762 from NIH, entitled "iCare Stress Management e-Training for Dementia Family Caregivers," to Bruno Kajiyama.

Table of Contents:

iCare Express: Background Information

The following guide is based on the *iCare Handbook*, which is created to go hand-in-hand with the iCare video training for caregivers of older adults with Alzheimer's or dementia. The *iCare Express* gives you quick access to the most frequently used forms from the video training program.

This is not intended to replace the complete *iCare Handbook*. Please see the *iCare Handbook* for detailed explanation and more information including examples, resources, and glossary of helpful words.

For more information, please visit: **www.icarefamily.com**

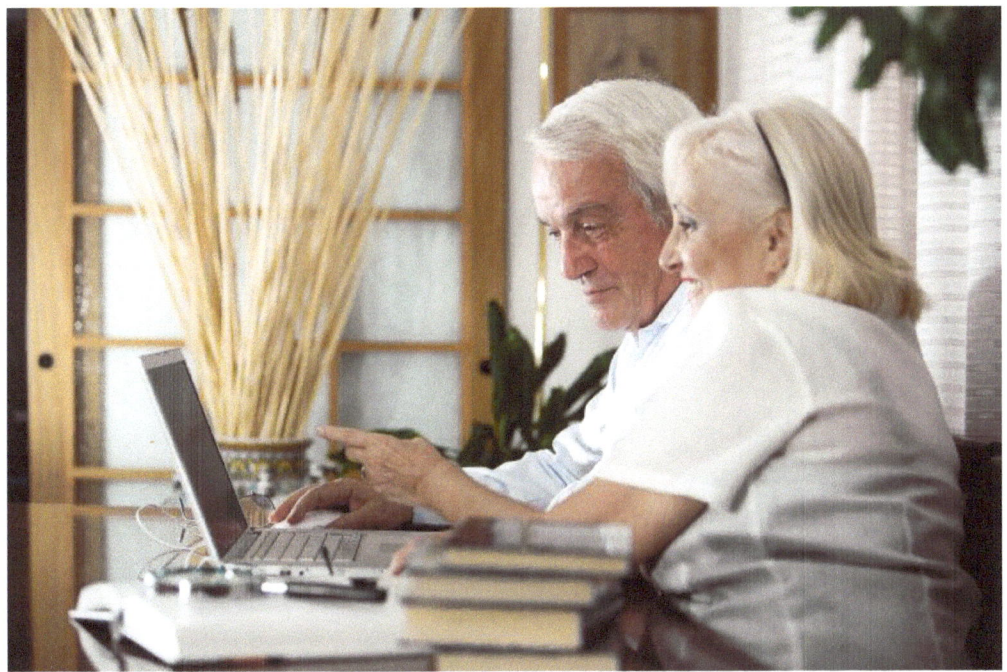

My Action Plan
Instructions

The "Action Plan" sheet is a tool for you to develop your own plan for the future after you finish each iCare training section. It's designed for helping you to process what you just learned in the training and how to implement the new skills in your unique situation in the future.

Each section of the sheet provides the space to write down your thoughts.

Review *(what did I learn in this chapter?)*
What you learned from the training you just completed. Was there new information to understand your situation? Perhaps a tool to improve your caregiving abilities?

Goal *(what do I want to accomplish?)*
What kind of new/different outcome you want to get.

Problems *(what might get in the way?)*
What can be the possible challenges to achieve the goal.

Solutions *(how to work around problems?)*
Brainstorm possible solutions to go around the problems for achieving the goal.

I can do it *(rate your confidence level)*
How confident are you from 1-*"definitely not "*to 10-*"definitely yes"*? If it is low, what do you need to make you feel more confident?

Actions *(what needs to be done, how, when, where, etc.)*
Write down a detailed action plan to achieve the goal in your situation.

Come back to your Action Plan after one to two weeks and check your progress.

Notes *(what worked? what did not work? how can it be improved?)*
Commend yourself for making positive action changes. If the plan is not working well to improve the situation, you can adjust your plan with different actions.

This is a tool to help you, not a test to put you down. Go easy and don't expect to do perfectly from the beginning. You do not need to be discouraged if the original plan is not working after a while. Just make a small change to try a different way.

My Action Plan

Review *(what did I learn in this chapter?)*

Goal *(what do I want to accomplish?)*

Problems *(what might get in the way?)*	Solutions *(how to work around problems)*

I can do it *(rate your confidence level)*

Definitely Not					Maybe				Definitely Yes
1	2	3	4	5	6	7	8	9	10

Actions *(what needs to be done, how, when, where, etc.)*

Save this for follow up later (aim for within one to two weeks)

Notes *(What worked? What did not work? How can it be improved?)*

The more you practice the skills, the more likely you are to feel better about yourself ☺

My Thought Record
Instructions
(From the iCare Handbook chapter - **Dealing with Stress**)

The *Thought Record* is a stress journal to reduce stress and improve your overall mood by challenging and replacing unhelpful thoughts. By completing this form, **you will learn to become aware of and monitor your negative thoughts.** This is a very useful way to reduce stress and improve your overall mood.

In the top box, **Situation,** briefly explain the stressful situation that occurred. Then, complete the columns one through five:

1. Current Thoughts
What were the first thoughts running through your mind when the disturbing behavior occurred?

2. Feelings
How did the situation make you feel? Were you sad, anxious, mad, or scared? There are numerous emotions, and now would be a good chance to reflect on how the disturbing behavior made you feel.

> **NOTE:** It's important that you make sure you aren't writing thoughts as feelings, or feelings as thoughts. These two concepts are not the same.

3. Challenge the thought
Ask yourself if your thought was completely true, or maybe there were exaggerations or miscommunication. Starting this by asking yourself:

"What is the evidence that the thought of __(enter your thought here)__ is true?"

4. Replacement (*What is a more creative or assertive way of thinking?*)
After you've challenged the thought, you can then replace the thought with a more accurate description of what happened and how you could have thought about or approached the situation (the approach will be noted in the next question below).

5. Future Actions *(How will I react differently next time?)*
Now you understand how your feelings can affect thoughts, and how you can challenge and replace them with more creative thoughts. Let's plan so you can respond differently in the future.

My Thought Record

Situation:

1. Current Thoughts	2. Feelings	3. Challenge the Thought	4. Replacement *What is a more creative or assertive way of thinking?*	5. Future Actions *How will I react differently next time?*

Pleasant Activities Log
Instructions
(From the handbook chapter - **Pleasant Activities**)

Taking time for yourself is important! It's not easy finding the time to do things you enjoy, but it's crucial to take care of yourself with pleasant activities so you don't get burned out or feel overly frustrated.

The *Pleasant Activity log* is a list of activities that helps you organize and add some pleasure to your everyday life.

1. Choose Pleasant Activities: Which events may you enjoy? Write down the "top ten" in the form. If you have difficulty finding ten, list five or six.

Tips to follow in making your list:

Tip #1: Start small and be simple. The most important thing to remember is to choose events that you can do every day or a few times a week. Choosing small events that don't require a lot of planning is the best way to start increasing pleasure in your life.

Tip #2: Choose events that you can increase. If you choose an event that already happens frequently, you won't be able to increase the number of times the event occurs. Focus on events you want to do more often.

---

2. Think and make a plan: Think about obstacles that will get in the way of your doing each event, such as:

- How am I going to find the time?
- I'll need someone to stay with my loved one while I'm out.
- I need money to *treat* myself

* Look at how you could possibly resolve these issues, because you may be disappointed if you can't do your event. Consider other Pleasant Activities, if needed.

* Use the *"Nuts and Bolts" of Pleasant Activities - Pleasant Activities Worksheet for YOU* (next page) to plan for each activity.

3. Fine-Tune It! You can hang this schedule somewhere you will see it every day, like the refrigerator, bathroom mirror or bedside table. It can remind you to do pleasant things for yourself throughout the week.

Place a check mark for each event after doing it on your *Pleasant Activities Log* and write the experience down to find out what went well and do it again.

After you try this, you can either revise your list and your plan, or if you are having success, continue to do what you are doing

Pleasant Activities Log

- List **Pleasant Activities** that you plan to do this week.
- Place a check mark next to each activity that you tried.
- Count how many activities you did each day.

Pleasant Activities	Mon __/__	Tue __/__	Wed __/__	Thu __/__	Fri __/__	Sat __/__	Sun __/__
1.							
2.							
3.							
4.							
5.							
6.							
7.							
8							
9.							
10.							
Totals for each day:							

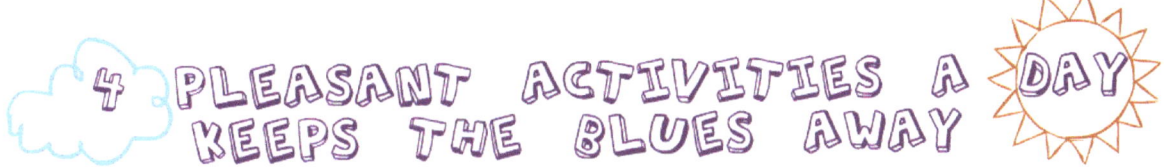

4 PLEASANT ACTIVITIES A DAY KEEPS THE BLUES AWAY

The "Nuts and Bolts" of Pleasant Activities Instructions

(From the iCare Handbook chapter - **Pleasant Activities**)

The "Nuts and Bolts" of Pleasant Activities goes hand-in-hand with the *Pleasant Activities Log* on the previous page. This sheet will help you to plan for your pleasant activity.

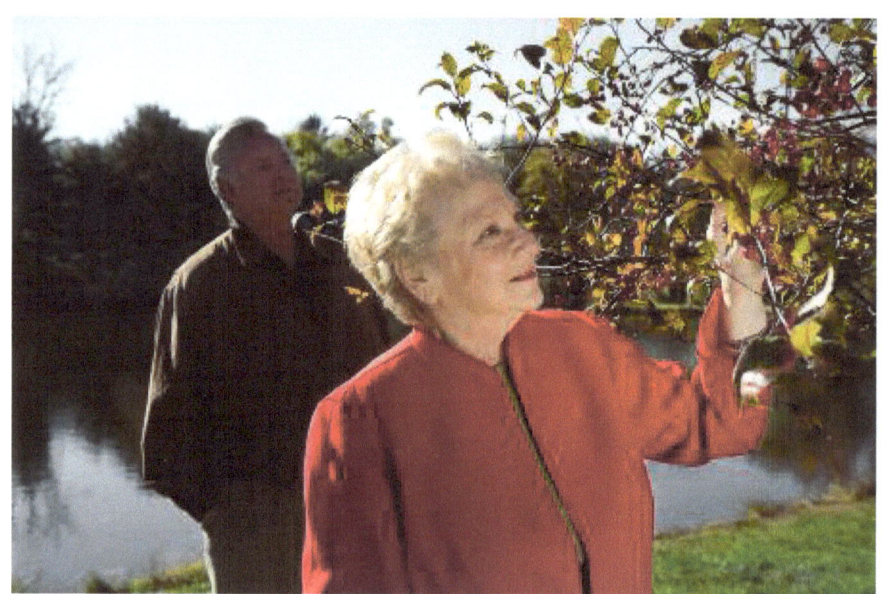

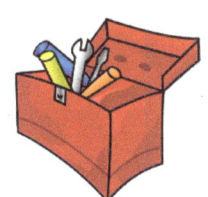

The "Nuts and Bolts" of Pleasant Activities

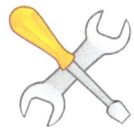

As we mentioned during the Pleasant Activities Plan, the idea is to commit to doing something for yourself on a regular basis. An excellent way to plan anything is to write out what you plan on doing and how you plan to do it. To help you in planning out your activity, we have provided a Nuts and Bolts of Pleasant Activities worksheet below. Please use this for each activity you try out. This will help avoid disappointing results due to forgetting to bring something or not remembering a necessary part of that activity.

Happy Event:	
Where?	
When? *(when, how often, how long)*	
What's needed? *(materials, things to bring)*	
How? *(arrangements and steps)*	

The "Nuts and Bolts" of Pleasant Activities
(For My Loved One and Me)
Instructions
(From the iCare Handbook chapter - **Pleasant Activities**)

The "Nuts and Bolts" of Pleasant Activities (for my Loved One and Me) goes hand-in-hand with the Pleasant Activities Log (for my Loved One and Me) on the following pages. This sheet will help you to plan for your pleasant activity.

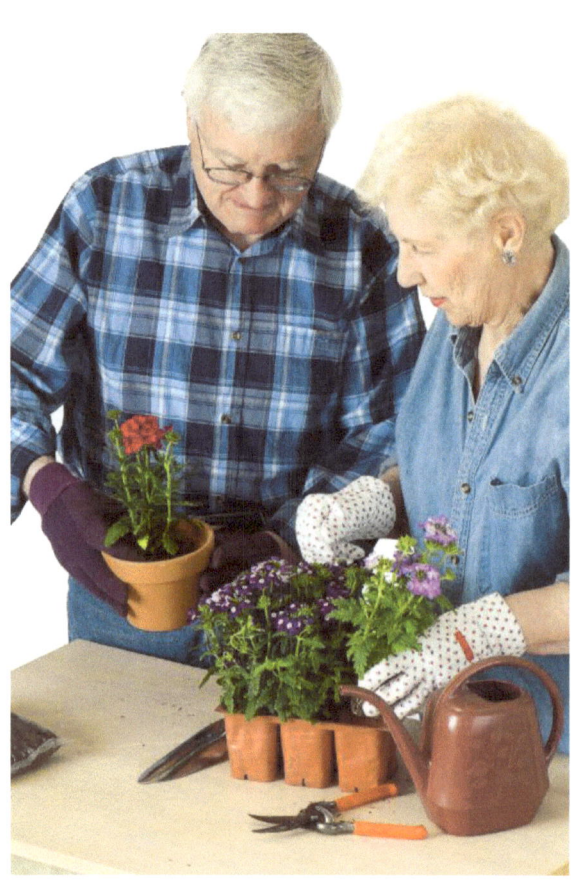

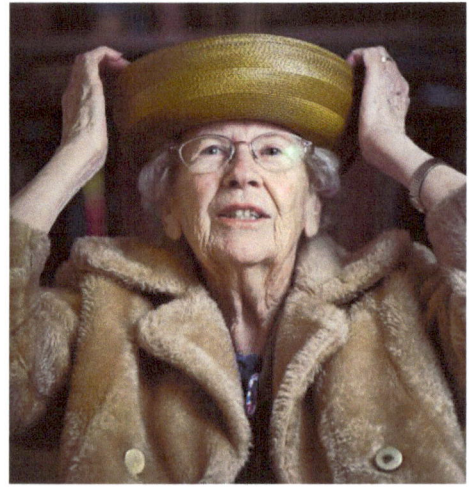

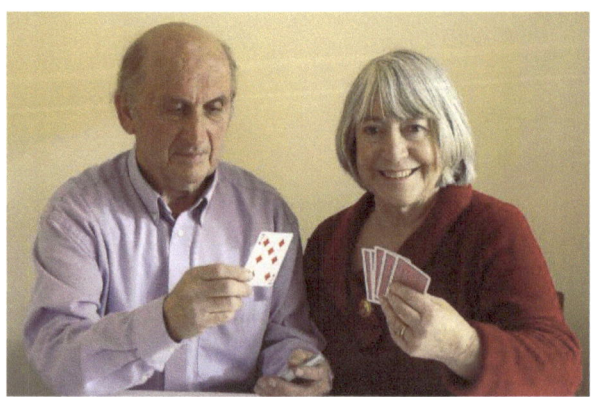

The "Nuts and Bolts" of Pleasant Activities
(For My Loved One and Me)

Pleasant activities can make the best use of a person's remaining abilities and can also reduce problematic behavior like wandering or agitation.

Because we want you to be successful in planning pleasant activities for both you and your loved one, we have put together a list of questions you should ask yourself beforehand so that things will go as smoothly as possible.

Think about the activity you have selected to enjoy with your loved one this week, and use the worksheet below to plan out your activity.

Happy Event:	
Where?	
When? (*when, how often, how long*)	
What's needed? (*materials, things to bring*)	
How? (*arrangements and steps*)	

Pleasant Activities Log for My Loved One and Me
Instructions
(From the iCare Handbook chapter - **Pleasant Activities**)

As a caregiver, it's not always possible to do things without your loved one. Your loved one also needs to be active and do things she or he enjoys. So it's important to try to do things together that you **both** enjoy. *Pleasant Activity log for My Loved One & Me* is a list of activities that help you organize and add some pleasure to you and your loved one's life.

1. Choose Pleasant Activities: Which events may you and your loved one enjoy? Write down the "top 10" in the form. If you have difficulty finding ten, list five or six.

There are some tips to follow in making and implementing your list.

Tip #1: Simplify the activity as much as possible: Start small and stay simple.
Tip #2: Don't force your loved one to participate: Encourage or reward him or her often.
Tip #3: Try to think of things that are similar to some hobbies, interests, or games your loved one used to enjoy.
Tip #4: Have a few activities available so if he or she becomes bored you can switch.
Tip #5: Plan to do activities in short bursts and match with your loved ones ability.
Tip #6: Try to involve other friends or family if at all possible.

2. Think and make a plan: Think about obstacles that will get in the way of your doing each event. Is your loved one able to do the activity alone or do they need help?

Look at how you could possibly resolve these issues, because you may be disappointed if you can't do your event. Consider other pleasant activities, if needed.

Use the *"Nuts and Bolts" of Pleasant Activities for My Loved One & Me* (previous page) to plan for each activity.

3. Fine-Tune It! Hang this schedule where you will see it every day, like the refrigerator, bathroom mirror, or bedside table. It can remind you to do pleasant things throughout the week.

Place a check mark for each event after doing it on your *Pleasant Activities Log* and write the experience down to find out what went well and do it again.

After you try this, you can either revise your list and your plan, or if you are having success, continue to do what you are doing.

Pleasant Activities Log for
My Loved One and Me

- List **Pleasant Activities** that you plan to do with your loved one this week.
- Place a check mark next to each activity that you tried.
- Count how many activities you did each day.

Pleasant Activities	Mon _/_	Tue _/_	Wed _/_	Thu _/_	Fri _/_	Sat _/_	Sun _/_
1.							
2.							
3.							
4.							
5.							
6.							
7.							
8.							
9.							
10.							
Totals for each day:							

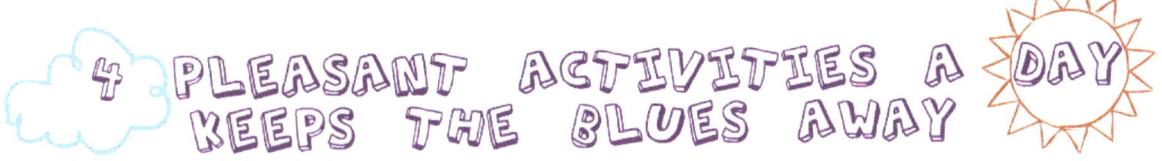

4 PLEASANT ACTIVITIES A DAY
KEEPS THE BLUES AWAY

Communication Check Sheet
Instructions
(From the iCare Handbook chapter - **Communication**)

Communication changes in persons with dementia. Learning new communication skills helps effective interactions and minimizes stress for everyone. This sheet helps you to be aware of how you communicated with your loved one this week, both verbally and nonverbally.

Section A: How you are presenting yourself
Explain what actually happened. Who was involved? Was anybody else close by? How did you react to the situation? Write down what you said (verbally) or did (non-verbally) to communicate with your loved one.

Section B: What your approach is
Write down **(1)** what style of communication you used, **(2)** how it turned out and **(3)** how you felt about it afterwards.

It's important to pay attention to how you are presenting yourself to your loved one. People with memory problems are very sensitive to non-verbal signals, such as facial expressions, body tension and mood. Are you tense? Stressed?

(1) There are three types of communication styles in general:
- **Passive Communication**
-*"You can take advantage of me. My feelings don't matter; only yours do. My thoughts aren't important; yours are the only ones worth listening to."*
- **Aggressive Communication**
-*"This is what I think; you're stupid for thinking differently. This is what I want; what you want isn't important. This is what I feel; your feelings don't count."*
- **Assertive Communication**
-*"This is what I think. This is what I feel. This is how I see the situation. Your thoughts and feelings are also important."*

Which communication style did you use?

(2) Write down the outcome. How did it work?

(3) Write down how you felt abut the whole communication and the outcome. Do you like how it turned out? If not, what/how do you want to change?

Your loved one will pick up on your feelings. If you are gentle, you are likely to help your loved one feel calm. Understanding your communication style and feelings may improve your relationship with your loved one and reduce stress.

Communication Check Sheet

Take notes on how you communicated this week with your loved one—both verbally and nonverbally. **In Section A**: Explain what actually happened. In **Section B**: Write down: **(1)** what style of communication you used, **(2)** how it turned out and **(3)** how you felt about it afterwards.

Section A.

What I said or did to communicate with my loved one:

_____

_____

_____

_____

_____

_____

Section B.

Style of Communication Used	How it Turned Out	How I Felt
_____	_____	_____
_____	_____	_____
_____	_____	_____
_____	_____	_____
_____	_____	_____
_____	_____	_____
_____	_____	_____

Medication List for Doctor's Appointment Form
Instructions
(From the iCare Handbook chapter - **Communication**)

One main concern caregivers have is communicating with their loved one's doctor. Usually, doctors have very busy schedules, so be sure you allow him or her to focus on treating your loved one during your visit by being as prepared as possible.

This "Medication List for Doctor's Appointment" form helps you with managing your loved one's medications.

Write down **drug name, what it's for and what it looks like, the doctor's who prescribed the medication, dosage,** and **instructions** for each medication.

Please keep this list of your loved one's prescription <u>and over-the-counter medications</u> and bring it to each doctor visit. You can print out and take to your loved one's next appointment.

You may also want to bring the actual bottles of medication along.

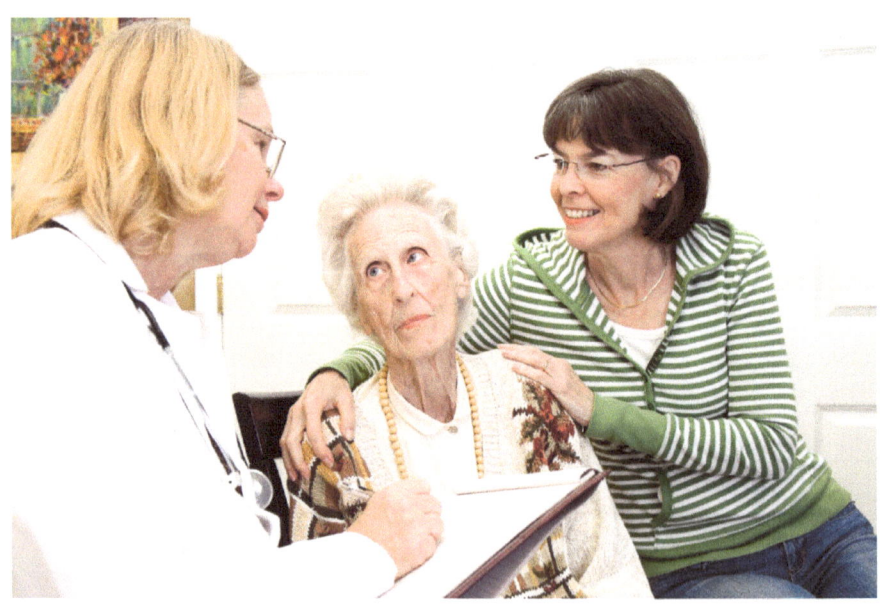

Medication List for Doctor's Appointment

Patient Name: _____

Drug Name	What It's for and Description of Pill (what it looks like)	Doctor	Dose	Instructions
Check with your primary doctor before stopping meds or taking any new medication from another doctor or a new over-the-counter drug.				

Medication List for Doctor's Appointment

Patient Name: _____

Drug Name	What It's for and Description of Pill (what it looks like)	Doctor	Dose	Instructions
Check with your primary doctor before stopping meds or taking any new medication from another doctor or a new over-the-counter drug.				

Doctor's Visit Worksheet
Instructions
(From the iCare Handbook chapter - **Communication**)

It's important to be aware of your loved one's current condition so you can provide effective and comfortable care. You can ask questions and develop a partnership with your loved one's physicians and the medical staff.

Often your appointment time is brief but there is a lot of ground to cover. It's a good idea to be well prepared before your next appointment or even before you call their office.

Please use "Doctor Visit Worksheet" to plan and focus what you want to discuss with his or her doctor effectively within the limited time. This worksheet helps you remember what you want to discuss.

Your list of questions needs to be short and to the point — for example, no more than two or three questions and write them in the **Concerns** section. You may want to advise the doctor early on in the appointment that you have some questions to talk about.

It's important that you become more familiar with all aspects of the "current problem" by writing it down in the **Notes** section:

*What, specifically, is the problem?

*When did you first notice it?

*How often does it happen?

*What seems to make it better?

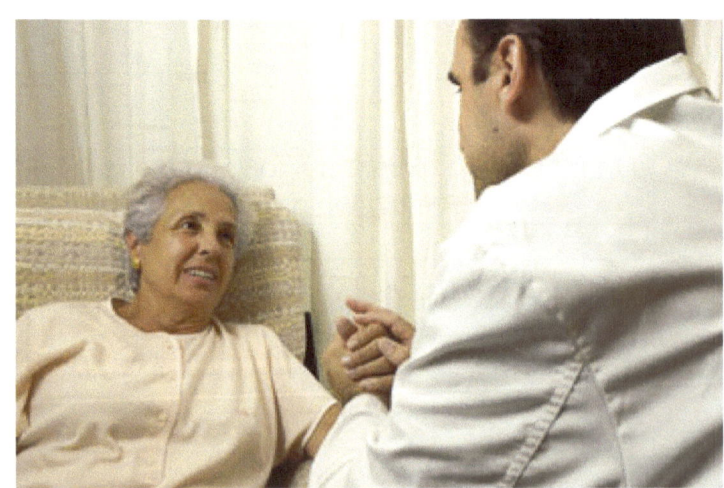

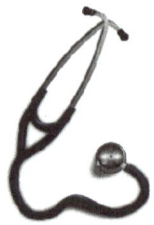

It's also a good idea to bring your *Medication List for Doctor's Appointment* (previous page).

Doctor's Visit Worksheet

Concerns: _____
1. _____
2. _____
3. _____

_____

Notes: _____

_____
_____
_____
_____
_____
_____

Doctor's Visit Worksheet

Concerns: _____
1. _____
2. _____
3. _____

_____

Notes: _____

_____
_____
_____
_____
_____

Trigger – Behavior – Response (TBR) Record Sheet
Instructions
(From the iCare Handbook chapter - **Managing Difficult Behaviors**)

A person with memory problems can no longer understand or engage in what is considered logical reasoning. So it is up to you to find ways to either change the "trigger" or your "response" if you want to manage the difficult "behavior."

This sheet helps you understand the situation and try to find out the causes or triggers that may explain why the difficult behavior happened. The behavior is more easily managed *after* changing the trigger and the response. Follow the direction below to fill out each sections after write down **date/day of week**, **time**, and **person(s) present.**

Note: With this worksheet, you start in the middle column with (1) Behaviors then work outwards to (2)Triggers, (3)Response, and (4&5)Strategies. The columns are numbered in the order you fill them in.

---

1. The problem behavior
List a difficult and challenging behavior your loved one does

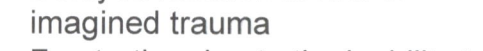

2. Identify the triggers
For people with memory problems, there are some clues or "triggers" that can explain their difficult behaviors such as:

- Physical discomfort (illness, medications)
- Drug interactions/dehydration
- Fatigue
- Loud noises or a busy environment
- Unfamiliar surroundings (new places, inability to recognize home)
- Complicated tasks, (activities or chores)

- Change in schedule or rushing
- Delayed reaction to real or imagined trauma
- Frustration due to the inability to communicate effectively, which may lead to depression

Understanding the cause of the difficult behavior is a key to avoid, manage or minimize triggers to improve the situation.

3. Your reaction/response to the behavior
Responses include what you do, how you feel or think, and what your loved one does. In other words, what happened *after* the behavior?

4. How you handled the situation
What kind of strategies you used to either change the trigger or your reaction for the situation.

5. Examine the outcome
Check out what worked and not worked. Commend yourself for partial successes and think about how you can improve the situation in the future.

T-B-R RECORD SHEET

Use this form to record what has worked and not worked when you tried to figure out how to better manage your loved one's behaviors.

INSTRUCTIONS: **1.** Identify the problem behavior. **2.** Think about the trigger—what led up to the problem behavior? **3.** Recall how you reacted/responded to the problem behavior **4.** Think of a strategy to try that will EITHER change the trigger or your reaction to that problem. **5.** Lastly, observe what happened after you used this strategy, and fill in the last blank.

Date/ Day of Week	Time	Person(s) Present	Trigger ⟶ Behavior ⟶ Response			The Strategy I used to Change the Behavior
			2.	**1.**	**3.**	**4.**
						What Happened after you used this Strategy?
						5.

21

Healthy Habits Thought Record
Instructions
(From the iCare Handbook chapter - **Healthy Habits**)

This sheet helps you to challenge and replace unhelpful thoughts, which may discourage you from starting more healthy habits. This is a modified version of the Thought Record (page 4) that can help you plan your healthy habits simply.

Below is an example scenario that uses the Healthy Habits Thought Record.

EXAMPLE SITUATION: We've been eating out/having fast-food lately because I can't find the time to prepare a nutritious meal for my loved one.

Column 1: Current Thoughts:
Ex: "I don't have the time or energy to prepare a nutritious meal for my family, so we're doomed to a fast-food lifestyle and obesity."

Column 2: How do you feel about that?
Ex: "I feel like a failure, tired, and unmotivated."

Column 3: What's keeping you from doing this differently?
Ex: "I don't know what to make. I don't have the ingredients when I do want to make something. By the time I get off of work, I don't have the time before my loved one is complaining of hunger."

Column 4: Brainstorm/ How could you make this work?
Ex: "I could prepare some foods ahead of time and put it in the fridge/freezer (like noodles and vegetables), and when it comes time to cook, just microwave/thaw, or toss them in what I'm cooking. I could take five or ten minutes to plan out our weekly meals and do little preparations like the refrigerator idea. Many sauces freeze well!"

Column 5: Goal for the next time:
Ex: "When my loved one goes to bed, I'll spend five to ten minutes making our weekly meal plan. I can wake up a little early for tiny preparations so that when I come home from work I can make dinner more quickly."

Healthy Habits Thought Record

(Thought Record for the Healthy Habits Chapter)

Situation:

Current thoughts	How do I feel about that?	What's keeping me from doing this differently?	Brainstorm: How can I make this work?	Goal for next time

Chart to Help Me Plan Healthy Meals for the Week
Instructions
(From the iCare Handbook chapter - **Healthy Habits**)

Being a caregiver, you have plenty of demands on your plate as it is. But taking care of yourself and finding the time and resources to eat a healthy diet shouldn't have to come last.

This "Healthy Meal Plan" chart can help you plan a week's worth of simple and healthy meals. Write down your weekly meal plan for breakfast, lunch, and dinner. You can use the chart to look at your diet and plan meals that are healthier and easier:

- prepare some foods ahead of time and put them in the fridge (ex: noodles, rice, boiled eggs, and vegetables)

- make a little extra to refrigerate/freeze for another meal (ex: soup, meatloaf, etc.)

- include a variety of food to get the nutrients you need.

- choose foods like vegetables, fruits, whole-grains and fat-free or low-fat dairy products most often.

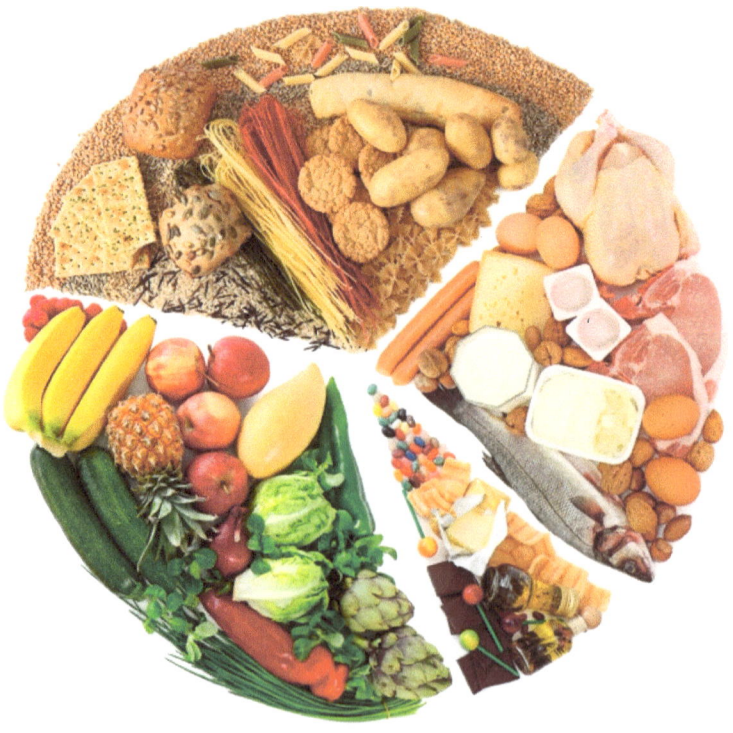

Chart to Help Me Plan Healthy Meals for the Week

Food for the Week

Dates: from _____ to _____

	Sunday	Monday	Tuesday	Wednesday	Thursday	Friday	Saturday
Morning							
Lunch							
Dinner							

DISCLAIMER:

Please be advised that the information being presented here is based on other research with distressed dementia caregivers in the United States. We do not know if it will be equally effective with all families in the United States or families living in other parts of the world since to our knowledge, information pertaining to this question is not yet available. Further, we do not guarantee or promise that the techniques illustrated in this training workbook (and related website and DVD) will be helpful to every individual caregiver who follows this training. For example, the problems you are confronted with may be different from the ones presented here, or you may have so many problems that you are overwhelmed and in need of professional assistance in order to cope effectively with your situation.

This training workbook/website/DVD is not intended to substitute for medical judgment as to the cause of your problems. Furthermore, it is not intended to treat any medical or psychological problems you may have as a family caregiver. This training workbook/website/DVD is an educational tool only, to help you and your family learn more about Alzheimer's disease and to give you information about common ways to cope with associated problems.

Individuals with medical conditions should not use the "deep breathing" or any of the other techniques presented here for stress management without their doctor's advice and approval.

Not all of this information is suitable for everyone. To reduce the risk of injury, consult your doctor before beginning this or any caregiver program. The instructions and advice presented here are in no way intended as a substitute for family counseling, psychotherapy, or any form of medical treatment. The creators, producers, participants, and distributors of this program disclaim any liability or loss in connection with the exercise and advice herein.